Vegan Soul Food Cookbook

Easy, Mouthwatering, Plant Based recipes for Everybody. Live Healthy and Longer with the Vegan Lifestyle

Isabel Underwood

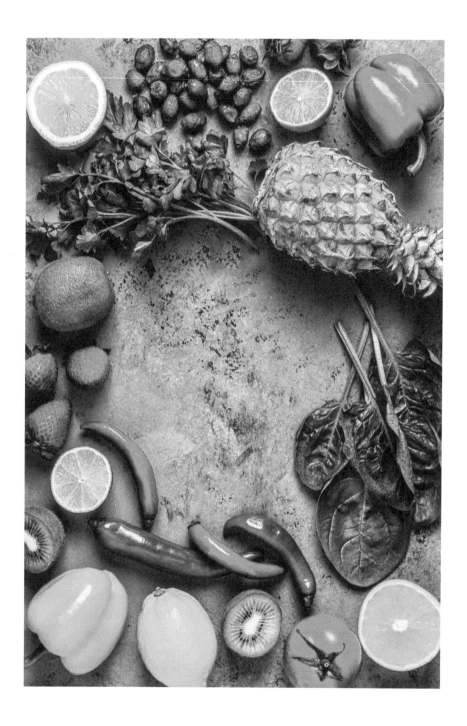

Contents

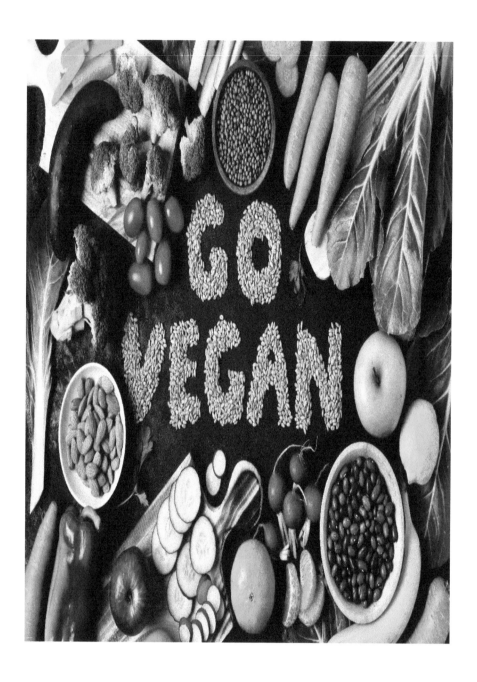

Vegan Cake with Pineapple and Mint

Prep Time 5 minutes
Cook Time 3 minutes
Total Time 8 minutes
Servings 4

Ingredients

4 slices fresh pineapple

2 ripe banana

2 tablespoons rolled oats

¼ cup cream of coconut

2 tablespoons quick-cooking oats

6 leaves fresh mint

½ teaspoon baking powder

2 teaspoons chia seeds

2 teaspoons poppy seeds

Directions

Combine pineapple, cream of coconut, banana, rolled oats, quick-cooking oats, mint, baking powder, chia seeds, and poppy seeds in a blender; blend until smooth. Pour into 2 mugs.

Microwave at the highest setting until mug cakes have set and risen well, about 3 minutes. Allow to cool a few minutes before serving.

Enjoy!

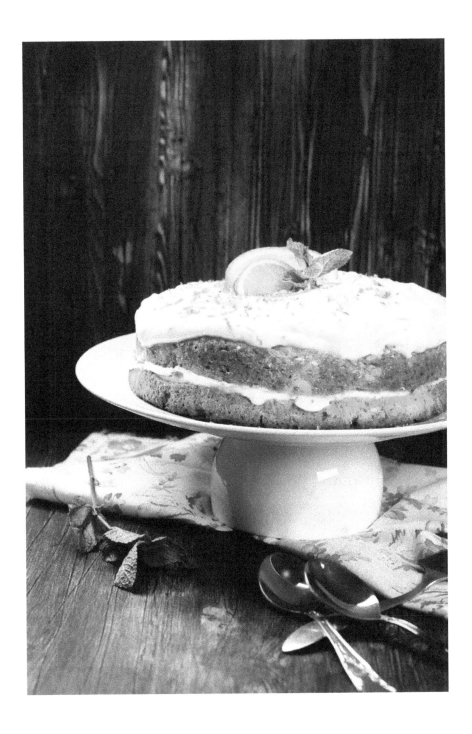

TOFU BREAKFAST BOWL

Prep time **15 mins**
Cook time **30 mins**
Total time **45 mins**
Servings **4**

Ingredients

¼ cup olive oil, divided

1 ⅓ (14 ounce) package extra-firm tofu, drained

⅘ teaspoon salt

2 teaspoons onion powder

2 teaspoons garlic powder

1 tablespoon olive oil

1 cups finely diced red onion

2 ⅔ jalapeno peppers, seeded and chopped

⅘ teaspoon salt

4 cloves garlic, minced

¼ cup chopped tomatoes

2 teaspoons cumin

1 tablespoon fresh lemon juice

1 ⅓ (15.5 ounce) can no-salt-added black beans, drained and rinsed

¼ cup cooked hash brown potatoes

1 ⅓ avocado - peeled, pitted and sliced

1 teaspoon fresh lemon juice

¼ cup chopped fresh cilantro

1 teaspoon hot sauce

black pepper to taste

1 tablespoon fresh lemon juice

¼ cup chopped fresh cilantro

⅘ teaspoon ground turmeric

Directions

Preheat a large, heavy skillet over medium-high heat. Add 2 tablespoons oil. Break tofu apart over skillet into bite-size pieces, sprinkle with salt and pepper, then cook, stirring frequently with a thin metal spatula, until liquid cooks out and tofu browns, about 10 minutes.

Add onion and garlic powders, turmeric, juice, and remaining tablespoon oil and toss to coat. Cook 5 minutes more.

Preheat a heavy-bottomed saucepan over medium-high heat. Add oil. Cook onion and jalapenos with a pinch of salt, stirring, until translucent, about 5 minutes, Add garlic and cook, stirring, until fragrant, about 30 seconds. Add tomatoes, cumin, and remaining salt, and cook, stirring, until tomatoes become saucy, about 5 minutes. Add cilantro and lemon juice. Let cilantro wilt in. Add beans and heat through, stirring occasionally, about 2 minutes. Taste for salt and seasoning.

Spoon some hash browns into each bowl, followed by a scoop of beans and a scoop of scramble. Top with avocado, a squeeze of fresh lemon juice, and a sprinkle of cilantro. Serve with hot sauce

Enjoy!

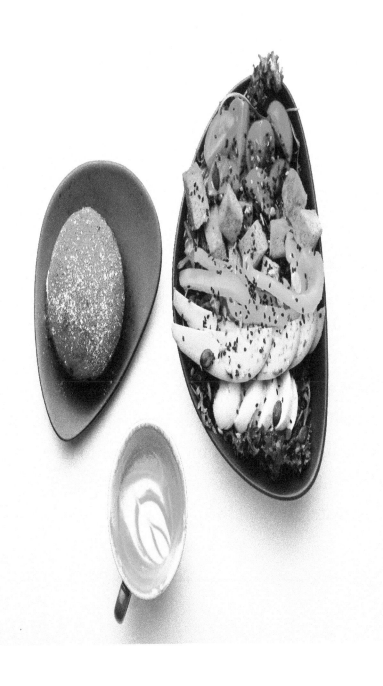

Zucchini Noodles with Chickpeas and Zucchini

Prep Time **10 mins**
Cook Time **15 mins**
Total Time **25 mins**
Servings **4**

Ingredients

½ cup olive oil

4 medium zucchini, cut into noodles with a spiralizer

4 cloves garlic, minced

24 zucchini blossoms, pistils removed, cut into strips

12 fresh basil leaves, cut into strips, or to taste

1 cups canned chickpeas, drained and rinsed

Salt to taste

Directions

Heat olive oil in a large skillet over low heat and cook garlic until softened, about 10 minutes.

Add zucchini and zucchini blossoms; mix well with olive oil. Add chickpeas and stir to combine. Season with salt and stir in basil.

Serve immediately. Enjoy!

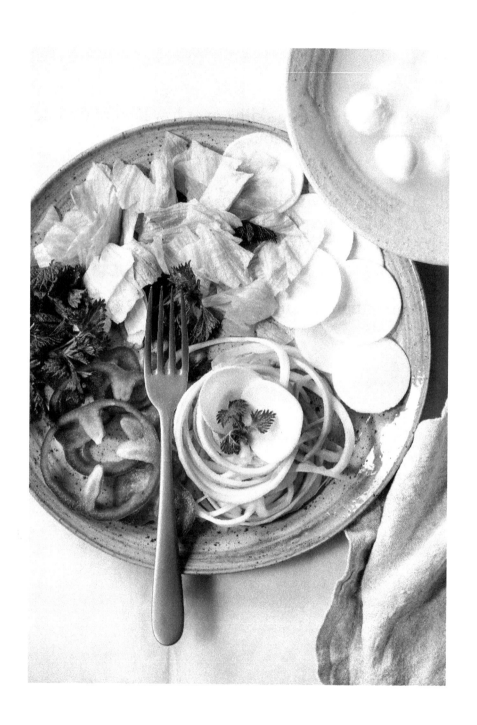

Couscous with Olives and Tomato

Prep Time **20 mins**

Cook Time **30 mins**

Total Time **50 mins**

Servings **8**

Ingredients

¼ cup and vegetable broth

¼ cup water

1 cups sliced black olives

½ cup couscous

2 pinch ground black pepper

½ cup olive oil, divided

1 cups pine nuts

8 cloves garlic, minced

2 pinch salt

2 shallot, minced

⅔ cup sun-dried tomatoes packed in oil, drained and chopped

½ cup chopped fresh flat-leaf parsley

2 cups vegetable broth

Directions

Bring 1 1/4 cup vegetable broth and water to a boil in a saucepan, stir in couscous, and mix in salt and black pepper. Reduce heat to low and simmer until liquid is absorbed, about 8 minutes.

Heat 3 tablespoons olive oil in a skillet over medium-high heat; stir in pine nuts and cook, stirring frequently, until pine nuts smell toasted and are golden brown, about 1 minute. Remove from heat.

Heat remaining 2 tablespoons olive oil in a saucepan; cook and stir garlic and shallot in the hot oil until softened, about 2 minutes.

Mix black olives and sun-dried tomatoes into garlic mixture and cook until heated through, 2 to 3 minutes, stirring often. Slowly pour in 1 cup vegetable broth and bring mixture to a boil.

Reduce heat to low and simmer until sauce has reduced, about 9 minutes.

Transfer couscous to a large serving bowl, mix with sauce, and serve topped with parsley and pine nuts.

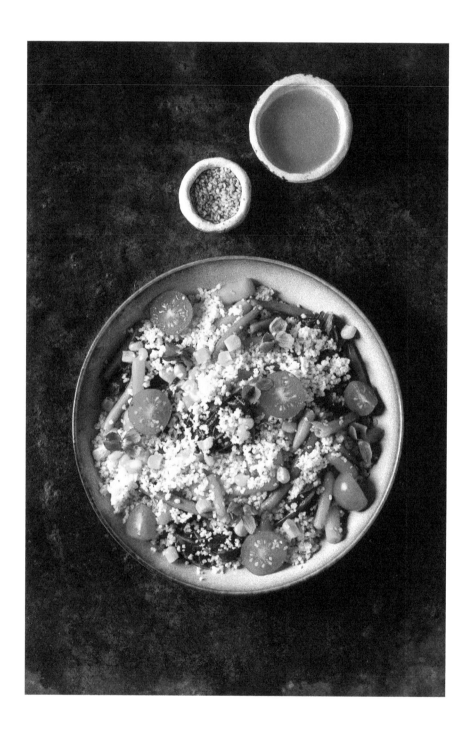

Easy Tomato Soup

Prep Time **10 mins**

Cook Time **45 mins**

Total Time **55 mins**

Servings **8**

Ingredients

¼ cup extra-virgin olive oil

8 cloves garlic, minced

2 onions, chopped

¾ cup cherry tomatoes, halved

8 tomatoes, chopped

4 bay leaves

4 sprigs fresh basil, divided

1 cup vegetable broth

Directions

Heat olive oil in a pot over low heat and cook onion until soft and translucent. Add garlic and cook until fragrant, about a minute.

Increase heat to medium, add all tomatoes, and cook until they start to break down, about 4 to 6 minutes.

Mix occasionally. Add vegetable broth, bay leaves, and 1 sprig of basil.

Bring to a boil, reduce heat, and simmer until tomatoes have broken down and soup starts to thicken, about 30 minutes.

Remove soup from heat and cool slightly. Remove bay leaves and basil.

Puree tomato soup with an immersion blender until smooth. Reheat soup before serving and garnish with basil leaves.

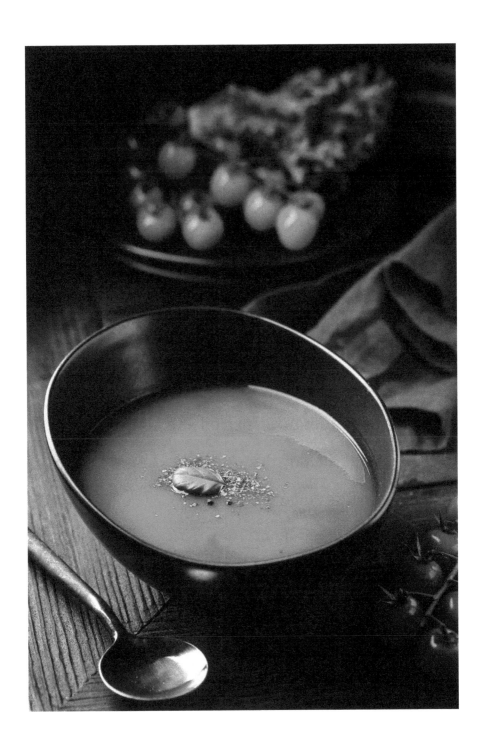

Italian Spaghetti Sauce

Prep Time **15 mins**
Cook Time **75 mins**
Total Time **90 mins**
Servings **4**

Ingredients

½ onion, chopped

2 tablespoons olive oil

2 pounds fresh tomatoes, peeled and chopped

¼ teaspoon garlic powder

1 teaspoon white sugar

1 teaspoon dried parsley

½ teaspoon salt

1 teaspoon dried basil

Directions

Heat olive oil in a large skillet over medium heat. Add onion and garlic powder; cook and mix until about 5 minutes.

Add parsley, tomatoes, basil, sugar, and salt.

Bring to a boil. Reduce heat and simmer, mixing occasionally, 1 to 1 hour and half.

Serve hot. Enjoy!

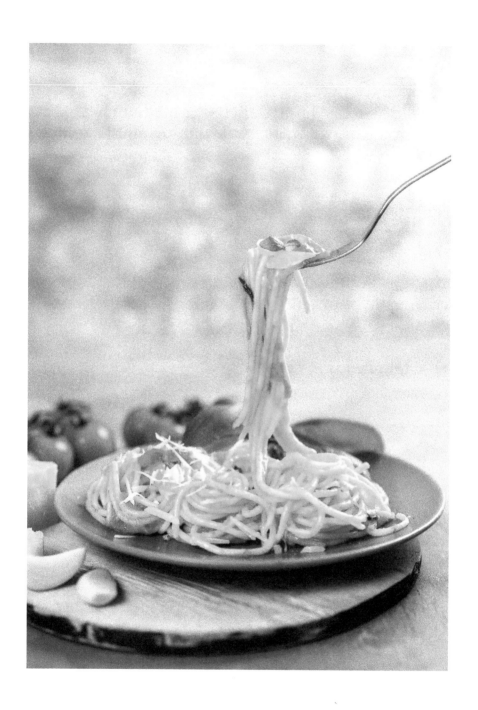

Delicious Brownies

Prep Time **30 mins**

Cook Time **50 mins**

Total Time **35 mins**

Servings **8**

Ingredients

2 tablespoons unbleached all-purpose flour

⅓ cup unsweetened cocoa powder

2 tablespoons white sugar

½ teaspoon salt

½ teaspoon baking powder

½ cup water

½ teaspoon vanilla extract

½ cup vegetable oil

Directions

Preheat the oven to 350 degrees F.

In a large bowl, stir together the flour, sugar, cocoa powder, baking powder and salt. Pour in water, vegetable oil and vanilla; mix until well blended. Spread evenly in a baking pan.

Bake for 26 to 30 minutes in the preheated oven, until the top is no longer shiny. Let cool for 10/12 minutes before cutting into squares.

Your Vegan Brownies are ready. Enjoy!

Easy Yummy Pancakes

Prep Time **5 mins**
Cook Time **10 mins**
Total Time **15 mins**
Servings **18 pancakes**

Ingredients

¼ cup and all-purpose flour

1 tablespoon baking powder

¼ cup white sugar

¼ cup water

1 teaspoons salt

2 tablespoons oil

Sift the flour, sugar, baking powder, and salt into a large bowl. Whisk the water and oil together in a small bowl.

Make a well in the center of the dry ingredients, and pour in the wet.

Mix just until blended.

Heat a lightly oiled griddle over medium-high heat. Drop batter by large spoonful onto the griddle, and cook until bubbles form and the edges are dry.

Flip, and cook until browned on the other side. Repeat with remaining batter.

Your easy, fast, delicious pancakes.

Vegan Muffins

Prep Time **20 mins**
Cook Time **20 mins**
Total Time **40 mins**
Servings **24**

Ingredients

2 cups brown sugar

¼ cup egg replacer (dry)

1 cups white sugar

½ cup all-purpose flour

4 large apples - peeled, cored and shredded

2 tablespoons baking soda

2 teaspoons baking powder

2 tablespoons ground cinnamon

1 tablespoon and 1 teaspoons salt

½ cup finely grated carrots

¼ cup and 1 tablespoon applesauce

½ cup vegetable oil

Directions

Preheat oven to 375 degrees F

Grease muffin cups or line with paper muffin liners.

In a large bowl combine white sugar, brown sugar, flour, baking powder, baking soda, cinnamon and salt. Stir in carrot and apple; mix well.

In a small bowl whisk together egg substitute, applesauce and oil. Stir into dry ingredients.

Spoon batter into prepared pans.

Bake in preheated oven for 20 minutes. Let muffins cool in pan for 5 minutes before removing from pans to cool completely. Enjoy!

Avocado Toast

Prep Time **10 mins**
Cook Time **10 mins**
Total Time **20 mins**
Servings **8**

Ingredients

8 slices whole-grain bread

1 teaspoons garlic powder

2 avocado, halved and pitted

¼ cup chopped fresh parsley

1 tablespoon extra-virgin olive oil

1 teaspoons salt

1 teaspoons ground black pepper

1 teaspoons onion powder

1 lemon, juiced

Directions

Toast bread in a toaster or toaster oven.

Scoop avocado into a bowl. Add parsley, olive oil, lemon juice, salt, pepper, onion powder, and garlic powder; mash together using a potato masher.

Spread avocado mixture into each piece of toast.

Serve and enjoy!

Blueberry Chia Pudding

Prep Time **10 mins**

Cook Time **8 h**

Total Time **8 h 10 mins**

Servings **6**

Ingredients

½ cup almond milk

⅔ cup fresh blueberries

¾ cup chia seeds, or more to taste

2 tablespoons maple syrup, or more to taste

2 pinch ground cinnamon

1 teaspoon vanilla extract

Directions

Combine almond milk, chia seeds, blueberries, maple syrup, vanilla extract, and cinnamon in a blender; blend until smooth.

Pour into 3 ramekins or glasses. Chill until set, 8 hours to overnight. Serve chilled.

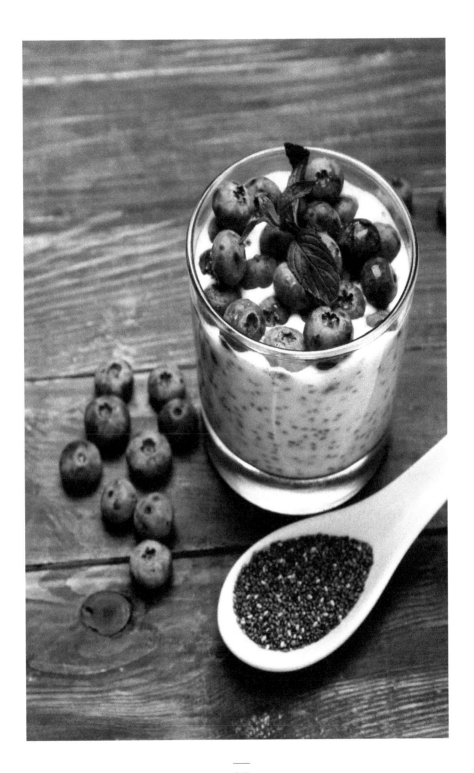

Banana Smoothie

Prep Time 10 mins

Cook Time 5 mins

Total Time 15 mins

Servings 4

Ingredients

4 banana

2 cups light unsweetened soy milk

1 cups chopped kale

1 tablespoon and 1 teaspoons maple syrup

¼ cup flax seeds

Directions

Place the banana, kale, soy milk, flax seeds, and maple syrup into a blender. Cover, and puree until smooth. Serve over ice!

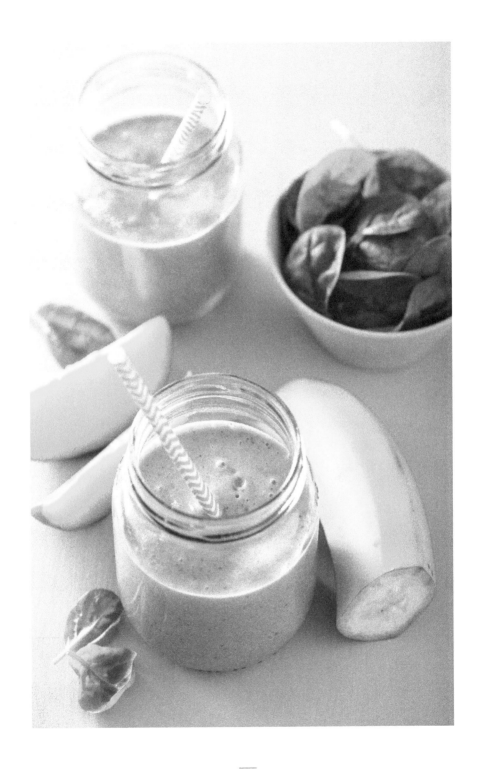

Vegan Crepes!

Prep Time **10 mins**

Cook Time **8 mins**

Total Time **18 mins**

Servings **6**

Ingredients

1 cups soy milk

½ cup melted soy margarine

1 cups water

2 tablespoons turbinado sugar

2 cups unbleached all-purpose flour

½ teaspoon salt

¼ cup maple syrup

Directions

In a large mixing bowl, blend soy milk, water, 1/4 cup margarine, sugar, syrup, flour, and salt. Cover and chill the mixture for 2 hours.

Lightly grease a 5 to 6 inch skillet with some soy margarine. Heat the skillet until hot. Pour approximately 3 tablespoons batter into the skillet.

Swirl to make the batter cover the skillet's bottom. Cook until golden, flip and cook on opposite side.

Enjoy!!

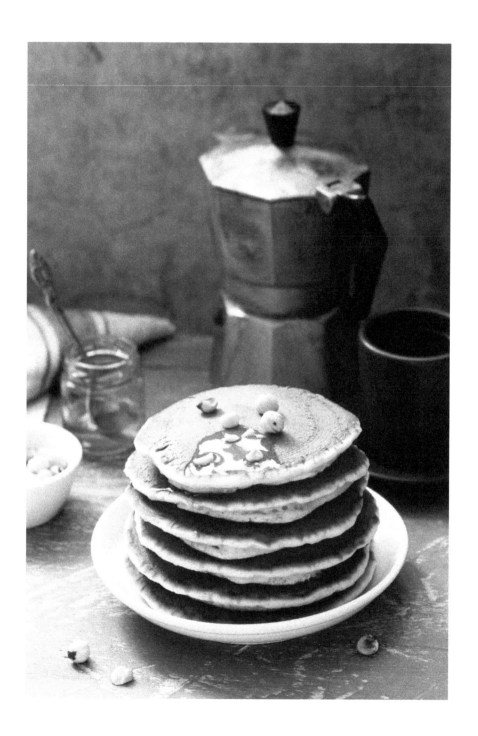

Quinoa Porridge

Prep Time 5 mins
Cook Time 30 mins
Total Time 35 mins
Servings 3

Ingredients

¼ teaspoon ground cinnamon

1 pinch salt

½ cup quinoa

1 ½ cups almond milk

2 tablespoons brown sugar

½ cup water

1 teaspoon vanilla extract (Optional)

Directions

Heat a saucepan over medium heat and measure in the quinoa. Season with cinnamon and cook until toasted, stirring frequently, about 3 minutes.

Pour in the almond milk, water and vanilla and stir in the brown sugar and salt.

Bring to a boil, then cook over low heat until the porridge is thick and grains are tender, about 25 minutes.

Add more water if needed if the liquid has dried up before it finishes cooking.

Mix occasionally, especially at the end, to prevent burning.

Easy Vegan Eggs

Prep Time **5 mins**
Cook Time **10 mins**
Total Time **15 mins**
Servings **8**

Ingredients

olive oil cooking spray

2 tablespoons nutritional yeast

1 teaspoons garlic powder

salt and ground black pepper to taste

½ teaspoon ground turmeric

¼ cup almond milk

1 teaspoons salt

2 (16 ounce) package firm tofu, drained and patted dry

Directions

Generously spray a skillet with olive oil cooking spray and heat over medium heat.

Add tofu, using your hands to crumble the block into smaller pieces; cook for 4 minutes.

Stir in nutritional yeast, 1/2 teaspoon salt, garlic powder, and turmeric.

Cook until seasonings have been incorporated, breaking tofu apart with a spatula to desired consistency, about 1 minute.

Stir in almond milk and cook until absorbed, about 2 minutes. Season with salt and pepper and serve warm.

Serve and enjoy!

Grilled Cauliflower Bites

Prep Time **15 mins**
Cook Time **10 mins**
Total Time **25 mins**
Servings **8**

Ingredients

1 large head cauliflower

1 teaspoon ground turmeric

1/2 teaspoon crushed red pepper flakes

2 tablespoons olive oil

Directions

Remove leaves and trim stem from cauliflower. Cut cauliflower into 8 wedges.

Mix turmeric and pepper flakes. Brush wedges with oil; sprinkle with turmeric mixture.

Grill, covered, over medium-high heat or broil 4 in. from heat until cauliflower is tender, 8-10 minutes on each side.

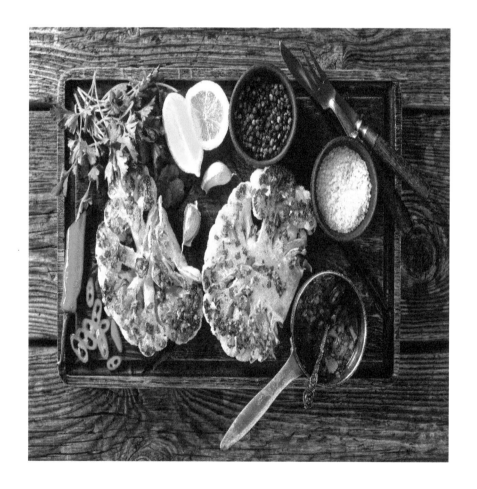

Stuffed Mini Peppers

Prep Time **10 mins**
Cook Time **10 mins**
Total Time **20 mins**
Servings **32 mini peppers**

Ingredients

1 teaspoon cumin seeds

1 can (15 ounces) garbanzo beans or chickpeas, rinsed and drained

1/4 cup fresh cilantro leaves

3 tablespoons cider vinegar

1/4 teaspoon salt

16 miniature sweet peppers, halved lengthwise

Additional fresh cilantro leaves

3 tablespoons water

In a dry small skillet, toast cumin seeds over medium heat until aromatic, 1-2 minutes, stirring frequently.

Transfer to a food processor. Add garbanzo beans, cilantro, water, vinegar and salt; pulse until blended.

Spoon into pepper halves. Top with additional cilantro.

Vegan Onions and Peas

Prep Time **10 mins**

Cook Time **10 mins**

Total Time **20 mins**

Servings **8**

Ingredients

2 large onions, cut into 1/2-inch wedges

1/2 cup chopped sweet red pepper

2 tablespoons vegetable oil

2 packages (16 ounces each) frozen peas

2 tablespoons minced fresh mint or 2 teaspoons dried mint

Directions

In a large skillet, saute onions and red pepper in oil until onions just begin to soften.

Add peas; cook, uncovered, stirring occasionally, for 10 minutes or until heated through. Stir in mint and cook for 1 minute.

In a large skillet, saute onions and red pepper in oil until onions just begin to soften.

Add peas; cook, uncovered, stirring occasionally, for 10 minutes or until heated through.

Stir in mint and cook for 1 minute.

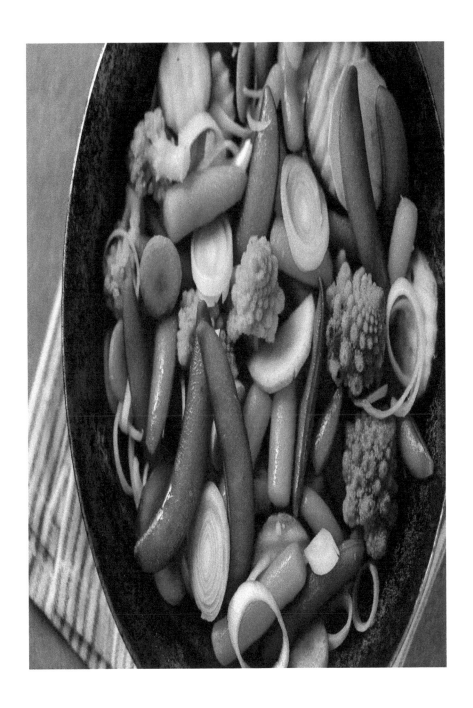

Tasty Roasted Chickpeas

Prep Time **10 mins**

Cook Time **40 mins**

Total Time **50 mins**

Servings **2**

Ingredients

2 cans (15 ounces each) chickpeas or garbanzo beans, rinsed, drained and patted dry

1 tablespoon chili powder

2 tablespoons extra virgin olive oil

1 teaspoon grated lime zest

2 teaspoons ground cumin

3/4 teaspoon sea salt

1 tablespoon lime juice

Directions

Preheat oven to 400°.

Line a 15x10x1-in. baking sheet with foil.

Spread chickpeas in a single layer over foil, removing any loose skins.

Bake until very crunchy, 40-45 minutes, stirring every 15 minutes.

Meanwhile, whisk together remaining ingredients. Remove chickpeas from oven; let cool 5 minutes.

Drizzle with oil mixture; shake pan to coat. Cool completely.

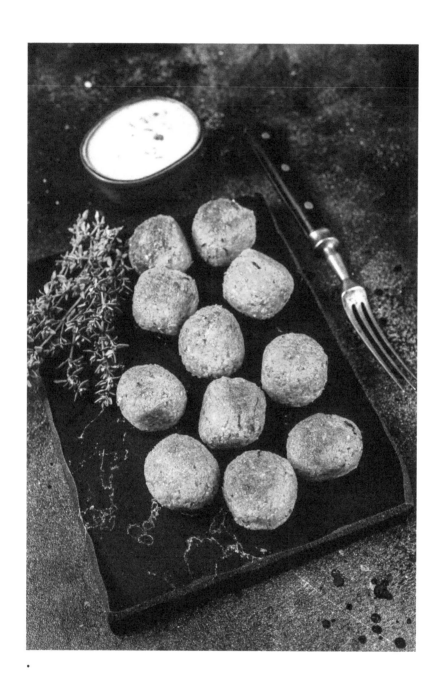

Easy Potato Chips

Prep Time 25 mins

Cook Time 5 mins

Total Time 30 mins

Servings 4 cups

Ingredients

7 unpeeled medium potatoes

5 teaspoons salt

2 quarts ice water

1-1/2 teaspoons celery salt

2 teaspoons garlic powder

1-1/2 teaspoons pepper

Oil for deep-fat frying

Directions

Using a vegetable peeler or metal cheese slicer, cut potatoes into very thin slices. Place in a large bowl; add ice water and salt. Soak for 30 minutes.

Drain potatoes; place on paper towels and pat dry. In a small bowl, combine the garlic powder, celery salt and pepper; set aside.

In a cast-iron or other heavy skillet, heat 1-1/2 in. oil to 375°. Fry potatoes in batches until golden brown, 3-4 minutes, stirring frequently.

Remove with a slotted spoon; drain on paper towels. Immediately sprinkle with seasoning mixture.

Enjoy!

Green Salad with garlic

Prep Time **15 mins**
Cook Time **0 mins**
Total Time **15 mins**
Servings **4**

Ingredients

1 pound kale, trimmed and torn

1/4 cup chopped oil-packed sun-dried tomatoes

2 tablespoons olive oil

5 garlic cloves, minced

1/4 teaspoon salt

2 tablespoons minced fresh parsley

Directions

In a stockpot, bring 1 in. of water to a boil. Add kale; cook, covered, 10-15 minutes or until tender.

Remove with a slotted spoon; discard cooking liquid.

In same pot, heat oil over medium heat.

Add tomatoes and garlic; cook and stir 1 minute.

Add kale, parsley and salt; heat through, stirring occasionally.

Fast Cilantro Potatoes

Prep Time **15 mins**
Cook Time **20 mins**
Total Time **35 mins**
Servings **8**

Ingredients

1 bunch fresh cilantro, chopped

1 garlic clove, minced

1/4 cup olive oil

3 pounds potatoes, peeled and cubed

1/2 teaspoon salt

Directions

In a large cast-iron or other heavy skillet, cook cilantro and garlic in oil over medium heat for 1 minute. Add the potatoes; cook and stir until tender and lightly browned, 20-25 minutes. Drain. Sprinkle with salt.

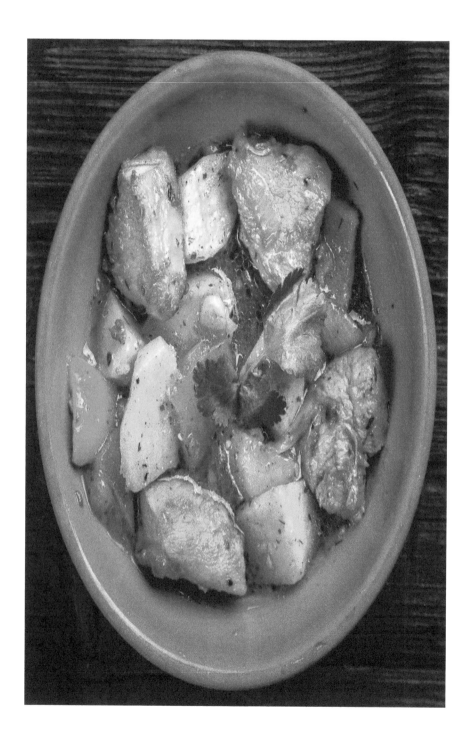

Garlic Mushrooms

Prep Time **15 mins**

Cook Time **15 mins**

Total Time **30 mins**

Servings **2**

Ingredients

1/4 cup lemon juice

2 tablespoons olive oil

3 tablespoons minced fresh parsley

Pepper to taste

3 garlic cloves, minced

1 pound large fresh mushrooms

Directions

For dressing, whisk together first 5 ingredients. Toss mushrooms with 2 tablespoons dressing.

Grill mushrooms, covered, over medium-high heat until tender, 5-7 minutes per side.

Mix with remaining dressing before serving.

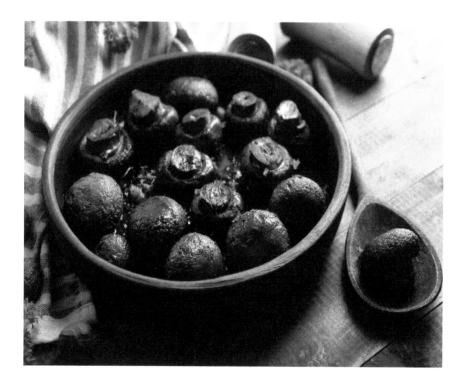

Roasted Asparagus

Prep Time **15 mins**

Cook Time **20 mins**

Total Time **35 mins**

Servings **12**

Ingredients

12 medium leeks (white portion only), halved lengthwise

3 pounds fresh asparagus, trimmed

1-1/2 teaspoons dill weed

1/2 teaspoon crushed red pepper flakes

1/4 teaspoon pepper

1/2 teaspoon salt

4-1/2 teaspoons olive oil

Place asparagus and leeks on an ungreased 15x10x1-in. baking pan.

Combine the remaining ingredients; pour over vegetables.

Bake at 400° for 20-25 minutes or until tender, stirring occasionally.

Enjoy!

Delicious Grilled Eggplant

Prep Time **15 mins**
Cook Time **5 mins**
Total Time **20 mins**
Servings **8**

Ingredients

2 small eggplants, cut into 1/2-inch slices

2 tablespoons lime juice

3 teaspoons Cajun seasoning

1/4 cup olive oil

Directions

Brush eggplant slices with oil. Drizzle with lime juice; sprinkle with Cajun seasoning. Let stand 5 minutes.

Grill eggplant, covered, over medium heat or broil 4 in. from heat until tender, 4-5 minutes per side.

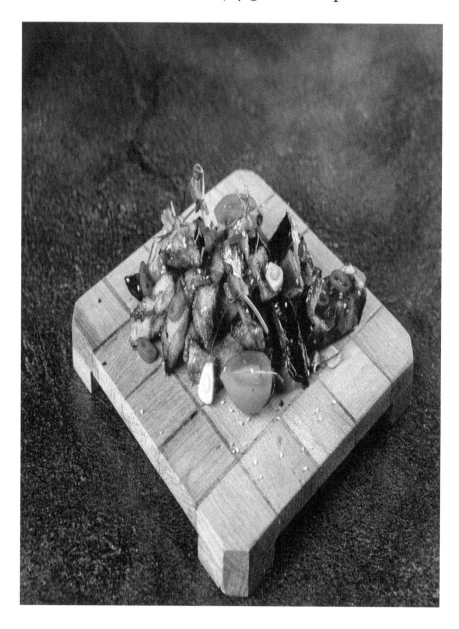

Easy Guacamole

Prep Time **10 mins**

Cook Time **0 mins**

Total Time **10 mins**

Servings **2**

Ingredients

2 medium ripe avocados

1 tablespoon lemon juice

1/8 to 1/4 teaspoon salt

1/4 cup chunky salsa

Directions

Peel and chop avocados; place in a small bowl. Sprinkle with lemon juice. Add salsa and salt; mash coarsely with a fork. Refrigerate until serving.

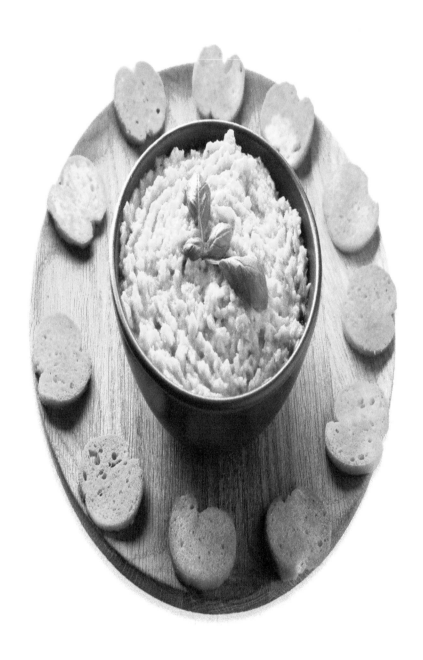

Zucchini Saute

Prep Time **10 mins**
Cook Time **5 mins**
Total Time **15 mins**
Servings **4**

Ingredients

1-pound medium zucchini, quartered lengthwise and halved

1 tablespoon olive oil

1/2 vegetable bouillon cube, crushed

2 tablespoons minced fresh parsley

1/4 cup finely chopped onion

1 teaspoon minced fresh thyme or 1/4 teaspoon dried thyme

Directions

In a large skillet, heat oil over medium-high heat.

Add zucchini, onion and bouillon; cook and stir 4-5 minutes or until zucchini is crisp-tender.

Sprinkle with herbs.

Summer Fruit Bowl

Prep Time **15 mins**
Cook Time **0 mins**
Total Time **15 mins**
Servings **16**

Ingredients

1 to 2 tablespoons corn syrup

8 cups fresh melon cubes

1 pint fresh strawberries, halved

2 oranges, sectioned

2 cups fresh pineapple chunks

Fresh mint leaves, optional

Directions

In a large bowl, combine melon cubes and corn syrup. Cover and refrigerate overnight.

Just before serving, stir in remaining fruit. Garnish with fresh mint leaves if desired.

Enjoy!

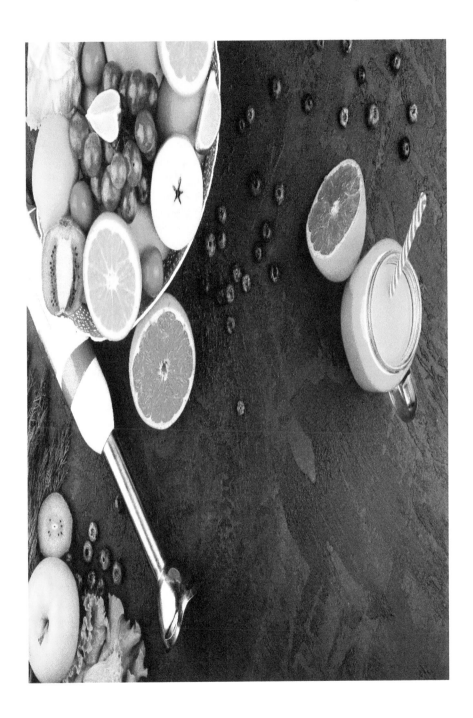

Vegan Baked Fries

Prep Time **15 mins**

Cook Time **20 mins**

Total Time **35 mins**

Servings **4**

Ingredients

4 medium russet potatoes

1 tablespoon olive oil

4 teaspoons dried minced chives

1/2 teaspoon salt

1/2 teaspoon garlic powder

1/4 teaspoon pepper

Directions

Preheat oven to 450°.

Cut potatoes into 1/4-in. julienne strips. Rinse well and pat dry.

Transfer potatoes to a large bowl. Drizzle with oil; sprinkle with the remaining ingredients.

Toss to coat. Arrange in a single layer in 2 baking pans coated with cooking spray.

Bake 20-25 minutes or until lightly browned, turning once

Enjoy!

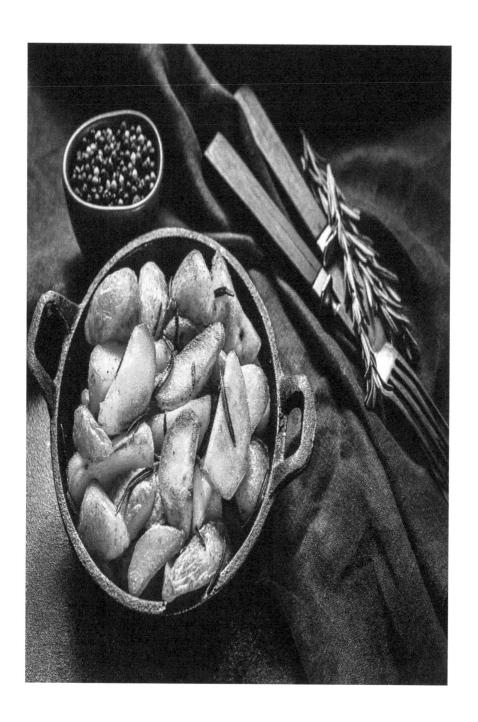

Garlic Brussels Sprouts

Prep Time **15 mins**
Cook Time **25 mins**
Total Time **40 mins**
Servings **8**

Ingredients

2 pounds Brussels sprouts (about 8 cups), trimmed and halved

1/4 cup olive oil

1 teaspoon salt

4 garlic cloves, minced

1/2 teaspoon pepper

1 cup breadcrumbs

1 to 2 tablespoons minced fresh rosemary

Preheat oven to 425°. Place first 4 ingredients in a small microwave-safe bowl; microwave on high 30 seconds.

Place Brussels sprouts in a 15x10x1-in. pan; toss with 3 tablespoons oil mixture. Roast 10 minutes.

Toss bread crumbs with rosemary and remaining oil mixture; sprinkle over sprouts.

Bake until crumbs are browned and sprouts are tender, 12-15 minutes.

Serve immediately.Enjoy!

Citrus Salad

Prep Time **15 mins**

Cook Time **0 mins**

Total Time **15 mins**

Servings **10**

Ingredients

1 pound medium jicama, peeled and cubed

8 tangerines, peeled, quartered and sliced

2 tablespoons lemon or lime juice

2 shallots, thinly sliced

1/4 cup chopped fresh cilantro

1/2 teaspoon pepper

1/2 teaspoon salt

Directions

Combine all ingredients; refrigerate until serving.
Enjoy!

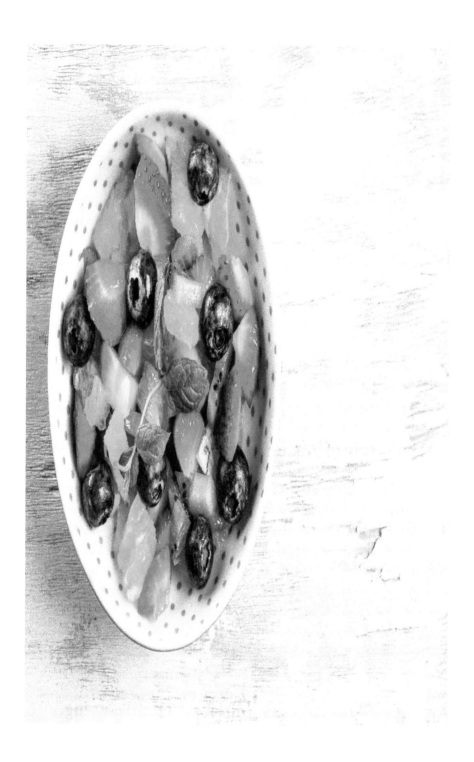

Cinnamon and Ginger Cookies

Prep Time **10 mins**

Cook Time **10 mins**

Total Time **20 mins**

Servings **12**

Ingredients

1/4 cup Almond Milk

1/2 cup vegetable or coconut oil

2 cups wholemeal flour

1 tsp baking soda

1 tbsp ground cinnamon

1 cup brown/coconut sugar

1 tbsp ground ginger

1/2 tsp salt

Directions

Sift the dry ingredients (flour, baking soda, cinnamon, ginger, salt & sugar) into a bowl and mix together.

Add the wet ingredients (almond milk & oil) and mix together until combined to form a dough.

Roll out 12 balls of the dough and place on a lined baking sheet with plenty of space between them.

Bake at 180 degrees for 10 minutes, then allow to cool on the tray

Enjoy!

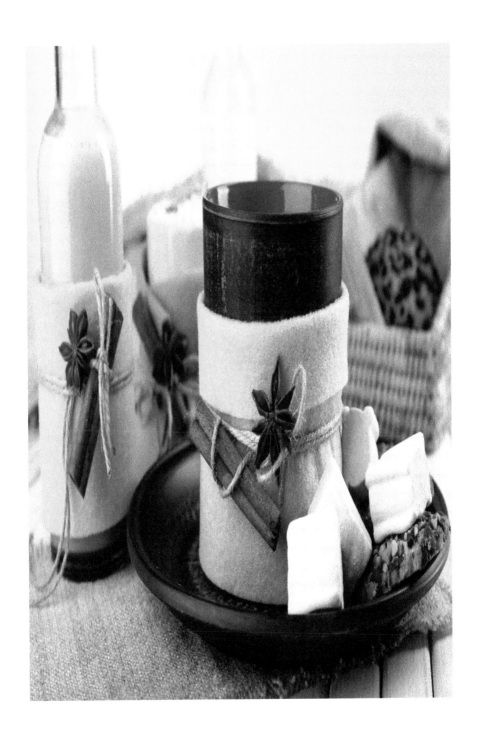

Delicious Tiramisu with Cherries

Prep Time 30 mins
Cook Time 30 mins
Total Time 60 mins
Servings 4

Ingredients

1 1/3 cup flour

3/4 tsp baking powder

1 tbsp cornflour

1/4 tsp sea salt

1/2 tsp bicarb soda

1/2 cup sugar

1/4 cup melted coconut oil

1 1/4 cup coffee-flavoured vegan milk)

2 tsp vanilla

1 can coconut whipping cream, chilled

Dark chocolate, shaved

1/3 cup cherry compote or cherry jam

Fresh cherries, pitted

Directions

Preheat oven to 340 degrees F.

Grease your cake tin with coconut oil.

Whisk together the flour, cornflour, baking powder, bicarb soda, and sea salt into a large bowl, set aside.

Add the sugar, melted coconut oil, and vanilla to a large bowl. Whisk to combine.

Add the dry ingredients to the wet ingredients and combine. Take care to not over mix. Pour the mixture into your cake tin.

Place in the oven for 30 minutes, or until a toothpick comes out clean. Let cool completely.

Cut the cake into circles the size of your serving glasses, set the excess cake aside.

Whip the coconut cream with handheld beaters. If using Full Fat Coconut Cream, scrape only the solid part from the top of the chilled can and discard the water before whipping.

Place the cake into the base of each glass.

Pour 2 tbsp of Califia Farms XX Espresso into each glass, infusing the cake.

Gently spoon in a layer of whipped coconut cream to each, then arrange halved pitted cherries around the outside of the glass.

Take the excess cake and crumble it into a bowl, place a couple of spoonfuls of this into the trifle glasses.

Top with cherry compote or cherry jam and dollop or pipe any additional coconut cream. Finish with shavings of dark chocolate. Enjoy!

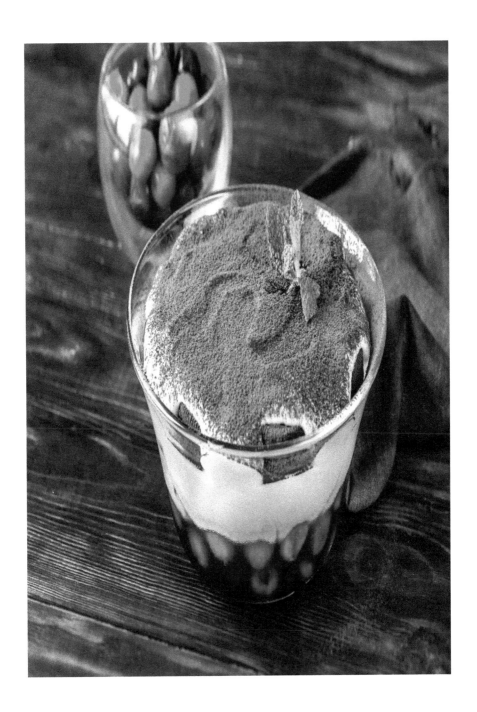

Vegan Double Chocolate Ice Cream

Prep Time 15 mins

Cook Time 5 mins

Total Time 20 mins

Servings 6

Ingredients

150g cashews

150ml warm water

3 tablespoons cocoa powder

1 tablespoon pectin

2 tablespoons cornflour

150g golden caster sugar

300ml coconut cream

200g vegan dark chocolate, broken squares

Empty the cashews, cocoa powder, warm water and pectin into a blender and blend on high until all is silky smooth. Pour into a large bowl and set aside.

Spoon the coconut cream into a medium saucepan and add the caster sugar and cubed dark chocolate. Heat very gently, regularly stirring until the sugar has dissolved and the chocolate has melted into the cream.

Measure the cornflour into a small bowl and add 2 tablespoons of the coconut chocolate mixture into the cornflour. Stir to combine until you have a thick, uniform, soft paste.

Return this paste to the saucepan and continue to stir until dissolved. Continue to cook the ice cream base for 5-7 minutes, over a gentle heat until steam rises from the mixture and the cornflour has performed its task and thickened the mixture.

The consistency will be that of double cream.

Pour the warm coconut and chocolate base into the cashew mixture and stir until thoroughly well combined.

Cover with cling film and set the ice cream base aside to cool.

Transfer to an ice cream machine and churn until frozen, about 45 minutes.

Transfer to a freezeable container and freeze overnight.

Remove from the freezer about 7/8 minutes before eating.

Enjoy!

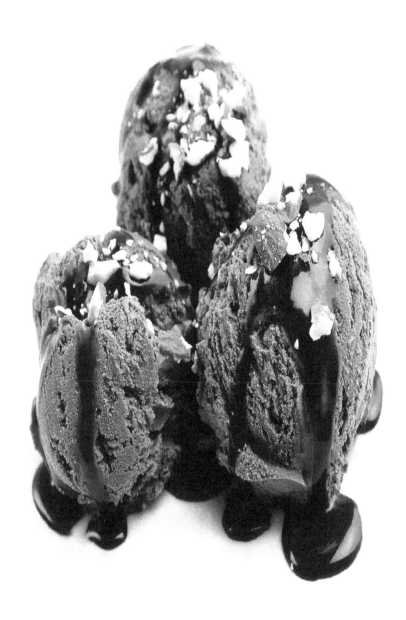

Pomegranate Cheesecake

Prep Time **90 mins**

Cook Time **0 mins**

Total Time **90 mins**

Servings **6**

Ingredients

For the crust:

300g vegan gingerbread biscuits

180g plant-based butter

¼ tsp salt

For the cheesecake:

2 packs vegan cream cheese)

100g canned coconut milk

2g agar-agar

2tbsp maple syrup

1 tsp vanilla essence

1 tbsp lemon juice

For the pomegranate syrup:

3tbsp corn-starch

300ml pomegranate juice

Pomegranate seeds to garnish

Directions

Place the gingerbread biscuits in a blender and blitz until they form a powder. Add in the butter and the salt and blitz again until combined.

Place in 6 individual greased tart tins and smooth over the base with the back of a spoon. Place in the fridge to set.

Meanwhile, in a small pot on low heat dissolve the agar-agar in the coconut milk, whisking constantly.

Once it comes to a boil, remove from heat and set aside.

In a large bowl mix the rest of the ingredients and slowly pour over the warm coconut milk, whisking until combined and creamy.

Divide evenly amongst the tart tins and place in the fridge for 4 hours.

In a small bowl combine 100ml pomegranate juice with the cornstarch. Place the rest of the juice in a small pot and bring to a boil for 5 minutes.

Pour in the cornstarch and pomegranate mixture and whisk for a further 5 minutes, until a syrup starts to form. Allow to cool.

Pour the pomegranate syrup on top and sprinkle with pomegranate seeds.

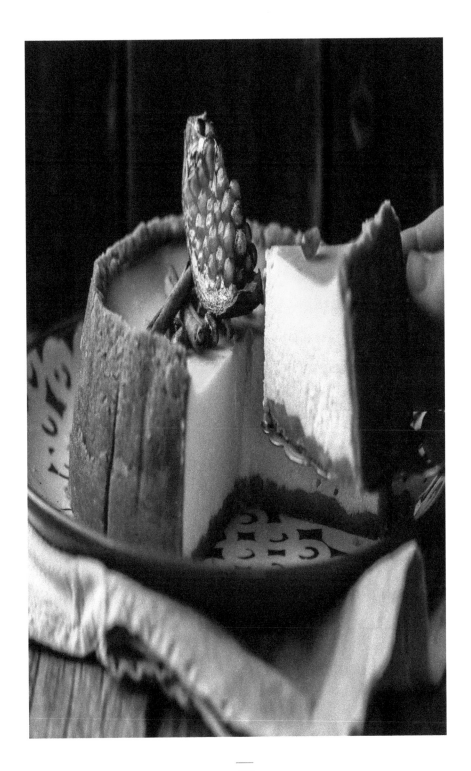

Vegan Brownies

Prep Time 15 mins

Cook Time 45 mins

Total Time 60 mins

Servings 10

Ingredients

390ml dairy-free milk

150g melted dark chocolate

50ml melted coconut oil

135g plain flour

90g Horlicks Vegan

50g coconut flour

50g cacao powder

80g light brown sugar

50g dark chocolate chunks

1 tablespoon of ground flaxseed

100g white chocolate chunks

Directions

Preheat oven to 360 degrees F.

Grease or line a rectangular baking tin with parchment paper.

In a large bowl combine the melted dark chocolate, melted coconut oil and dairy free milk.

Combine and then add the Horlicks Vegan, plain and coconut flours, light brown sugar, cacao powder and ground flaxseed.

Combine well and then fold 2/3 of the white chocolate and dark chocolate chunks through the mixture.

Pour the mixture into the tin and flatten so it's smooth.

Now scatter the remaining chocolate chunks on top and gently push down.

Bake in the oven for 40-45 minutes or until a toothpick comes out clean.

Allow to cool before removing from the tin, slicing and devouring!

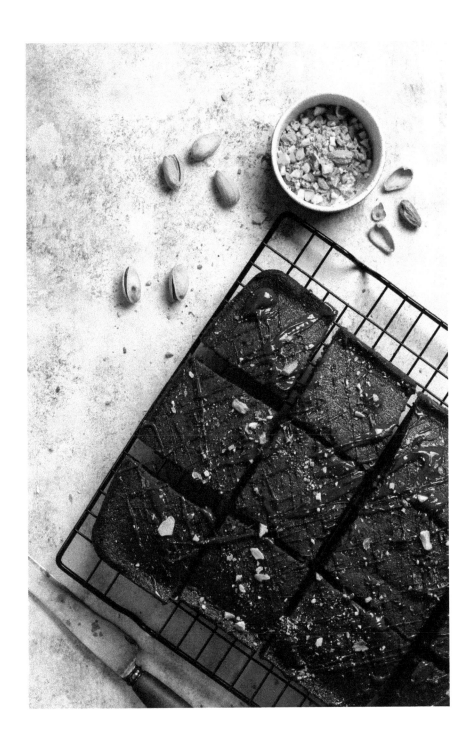

CPSIA information can be obtained
at www.ICGtesting.com
Printed in the USA
LVHW010403240621
690929LV00007B/835